Chair Yoga for weight loss Two in one

A Comprehensive Guide to Exercises, Mobility, and Weight Loss

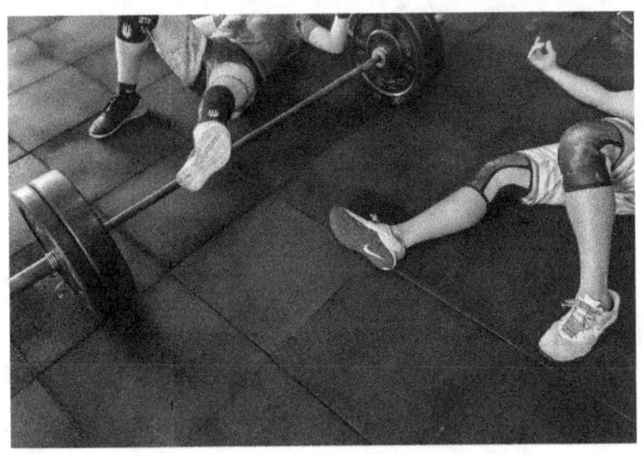

Dr. JERRY TAYLOR

Chair Yoga for weight loss Two in one

A Comprehensive Guide to Exercises, Mobility, and Weight Loss

Dr. JERRY TAYLOR

Copyright © 2024
By JERRY TAYLOR

All Rights Reserved.

However, most publishers and self-publishers include more information on their copyright pages for a variety of legal and business reasons. That's why using a copyright page template can help you make this process a whole lot quicker and easier.

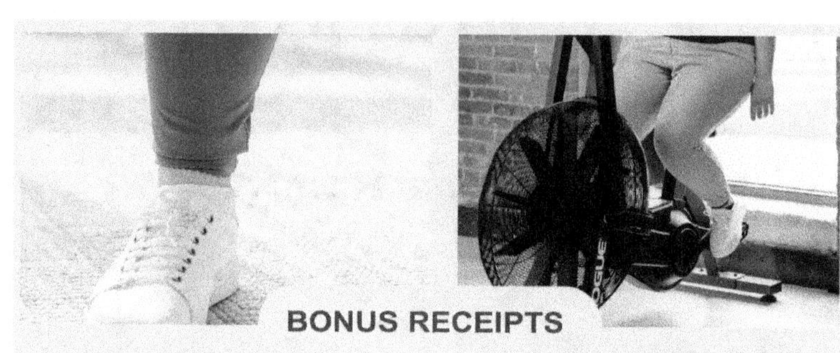

CHAIR YOGA FOR WEIGHT LOSS
TWO IN ONE

A COMPREHENSIVE GUIDE TO EXERCISES, MOBILITY, AND WEIGHT LOSS

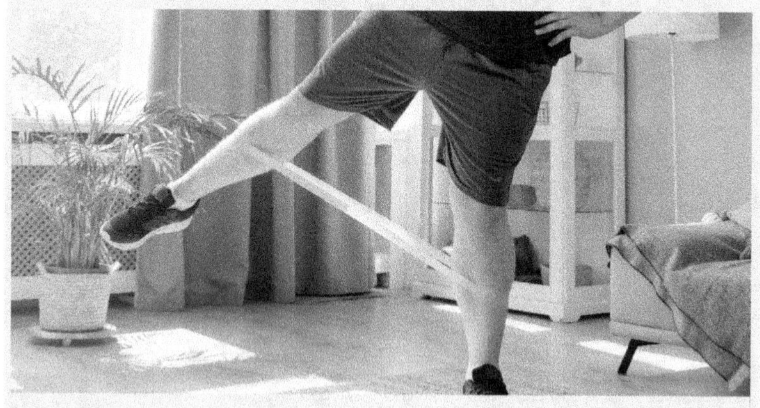

Description

Introducing "Chair Yoga for Weight Loss: Two in One"—your all-inclusive guide to achieving your health goals while harnessing the restorative qualities of yoga!

Discover the advantages of chair yoga, a mild yet effective form of yoga that blends the comforts of sitting with the well-known benefits of the poses. Anybody can benefit from this extensive e-book, regardless of their expertise level or mobility limitations.

Experience a sequence of challenging chair yoga poses that boost your flexibility, strength, and metabolism as you learn the secrets to reducing weight and exercising your body. Every programme, from targeted workouts to energising flows, is made to help you safely and effectively reach your weight loss goals.

In addition, "Chair Yoga for Weight Loss: Two in One" promotes not only your physical but also your mental and emotional well-being. Examine stress-reduction and inner-peace-promoting practices like mindfulness, breathing exercises, and relaxation approaches.

With its simple instructions, useful suggestions, and beautiful visuals, this e-book makes it easy to include chair yoga into your daily routine. Whether you're at home, at work, or on the go, yoga can help you whenever and wherever you are.

The first step to a better, healthier you is to read "Chair Yoga for Weight Loss: Two in One." Change your physique, reduce stress, and take up a lively, healthy lifestyle. Grab your copy right away to get going on the road to becoming a better version of yourself!

Table of contents

Introduction

Chapter 1: Understanding Chair Yoga: Basics and Benefits

What is Chair Yoga?

Origins of Chair Yoga

Benefits of Chair Yoga for Weight Loss

Chapter 2: Preparing for Chair Yoga: Setting Up

Chapter 3: Chair Yoga Pose: A Comprehensive Guide to Weight Loss Chair Sun Salutations

Chapter 4: Chair Yoga Exercises: Weight Loss Movements and Methods Morning Routine

Chapter 5: Chair Yoga Adjustments and Supplements: Tailoring Positions to All Ability Levels

Chapter 6: Breathing Techniques: Incorporating Pranayama for Improved Results

Chapter 7: Mindful Eating: Integrating Yoga Philosophy with Nutrition

Chapter 8: Combining Chair Yoga with Other Exercises to Create a Fitness Programme That Is Well-Balanced

Chapter 9: Tracking Your Progress: Setting Goals and Keeping an Eye on Outcomes

Setting SMART Goals

Tracking Your Progress

Adjusting Your Approach

Chapter 10: Frequently Asked Questions (FAQs) About Chair Yoga and Weight Loss

What is chair yoga, and how does it differ from traditional yoga?

Can chair yoga help with weight loss?

How often should I practice chair yoga for weight loss?

Are there specific poses or sequences that are best for weight loss?

Can chair yoga help with stress-related eating and emotional wellness?

Chapter 11: Bonus Recipes for Healthy Living

Chapter 12: Conclusion Thoughts: Chair Yoga - Embracing Well-being

Introduction

Welcome to "Chair Yoga for Weight Loss: Two in One"! I am thrilled to embark on this journey with you as we explore the transformative power of chair yoga for achieving your weight loss goals.

In this introductory chapter, I want to extend my warmest greetings to you and provide an overview of what you can expect from this unique approach to weight loss through chair yoga.
First and foremost, let me congratulate you on taking the first step towards a healthier, happier you. Embarking on a weight loss journey requires dedication, commitment, and a willingness to explore new avenues for achieving your goals. With chair yoga, we have a

powerful tool at our disposal—one that not only supports physical fitness but also promotes mental clarity, emotional well-being, and overall balance in life.

In "Chair Yoga for Weight Loss: Two in One", we will delve into the practice of chair yoga—a gentle yet effective form of yoga that can be adapted to suit individuals of all ages, abilities, and fitness levels. Whether you're a seasoned yogi or brand new to the practice, chair yoga offers a safe and accessible way to reap the benefits of yoga without the need for a mat or extensive physical exertion.

Throughout this e-book, you will discover a carefully curated selection of chair yoga sequences, breathing exercises, mindfulness practices, and lifestyle tips—all designed to support your weight loss journey holistically. From gentle stretches to dynamic flows, each practice is designed to engage your body, mind, and spirit, helping you build strength, flexibility, and resilience from the inside out.

But "Chair Yoga for Weight Loss: Two in One" is more than just a fitness program. It's a holistic approach to well-being that honors the interconnectedness of body, mind, and soul. As you embark on this journey, I encourage you to approach your practice with an open heart and an open mind, embracing the opportunity for self-discovery and personal growth along the way.

Living in the middle of a busy city's everyday bustle was a woman by the name of Maya. Maya, plagued by her hectic schedule and dealing with her weight, longed to find a way to prioritise her health without putting further strain on her life.

One day, Maya was looking through her phone when she came across a brand-new e-book called "Chair Yoga for

Weight Loss: Two in One." Maya decided to give the notion of combining yoga with diet plans a go because she found it intriguing.

As she turned the pages of the e-book, Maya entered a world of gentle movements and peaceful breathwork that she could practice in the comfort of her own chair. Maya was drawn to the relaxing rhythm of chair yoga, which included both simple stretches and more challenging poses modified for seated practice.

Maya dedicates a brief amount of time each day to her chair yoga practice, focusing on mental calmness and self-grounding. With every breath, her worry gave way to a feeling of brightness and lightness. But yoga wasn't the only thing that made Maya's life better. To help her with her weight loss, the e-book also offered sage advice on focused exercises and healthy eating habits. Maya began to gradually change her diet, eating her meals more slowly and including more fruits, vegetables, and whole grains.

Maya noticed a shift in herself as the days dragged into weeks. More than anything, she felt balanced, energised, and confident despite shedding pounds and inches. Her go-to strategy for dealing with stress and excess weight was a mix of chair yoga and diet plans.

Maya saw every day as a chance to better her body, mind, and soul, and she approached each one with a fresh sense of dedication and purpose. Maya has been able to find a truly transformative route to recovery because of the information in "Chair Yoga for Weight Loss: Two in One."

Maya discovered she was not travelling alone as she carried on with her journey. With the e-book as her roadmap and her faithful chair as her companion, Maya was ready to welcome a life of wellness, joy, and complete well-being.

Chapter 1: Understanding Chair Yoga: Basics and Benefits

Welcome to "Chair Yoga for Weight Loss: Two in One"! In this chapter, we will explore the fundamentals of chair yoga, its origins, and the myriad benefits it offers for weight loss and overall well-being.

What is Chair Yoga?

Chair yoga is a modified form of yoga that adapts traditional yoga poses and practices to be performed while seated on a chair or using a chair for support. It is an accessible and inclusive practice suitable for individuals of all ages, abilities, and fitness levels. Chair yoga incorporates gentle movements, stretches, and breathing techniques to promote physical, mental, and emotional health.

Origins of Chair Yoga

The roots of chair yoga can be traced back to the ancient practice of hatha yoga, which originated in India over 5,000 years ago. Over time, yoga evolved to accommodate the needs of individuals with physical limitations or mobility challenges. Chair yoga emerged as a way to make yoga more accessible and inclusive for everyone, regardless of age, health, or physical condition.

Benefits of Chair Yoga for Weight Loss

Chair yoga offers a multitude of benefits that can support your weight loss journey in various ways:

1. Low-Impact Exercise: Chair yoga provides a gentle yet effective form of exercise that is easy on the joints and suitable for individuals with mobility issues or injuries. The controlled movements and stretches help improve flexibility, mobility, and muscle tone, contributing to overall calorie expenditure.

2. Increased Metabolism: Practicing chair yoga stimulates circulation, enhances digestion, and boosts metabolism, which can aid in weight management and calorie burning.

3. Mindful Eating: Chair yoga cultivates mindfulness and awareness, helping you develop a healthier relationship with food. By practicing mindfulness techniques, such as mindful eating, you can become more attuned to your body's hunger and fullness cues, leading to better portion control and healthier eating habits.

4. Stress Reduction: Stress is a common trigger for emotional eating and weight gain. Chair yoga incorporates relaxation techniques, such as deep breathing and meditation, to promote stress reduction, mental clarity, and emotional balance.

5. Improved Body Awareness: Chair yoga encourages greater body awareness and self-acceptance, fostering a positive body image and mindset conducive to sustainable weight loss goals.

Chapter 2: Preparing for Chair Yoga: Setting Up

Welcome to Chapter 2 of "Chair Yoga for Weight Loss: Two in One". In this chapter, we'll explore how to set up your space and prepare yourself for a successful chair yoga practice. Setting the right environment and mindset is crucial for getting the most out of your sessions and achieving your fitness goals.

1. Find a Quiet Space:
Choose a quiet and clutter-free area where you can comfortably practice chair yoga without distractions. This could be a corner of your living room, a peaceful spot in your bedroom, or even your office during a break. Creating a serene environment will help you focus and fully engage in your practice.

2. Select the Right Chair:

Ensure you have a sturdy chair with a straight back and no armrests. The chair should be stable and supportive to accommodate various yoga poses and movements. Avoid using chairs with wheels or cushions, as they may compromise your balance during the practice.

3. Dress Comfortably:

Wear loose, breathable clothing that allows for freedom of movement. Choose attire that makes you feel comfortable and confident, whether it's yoga leggings and a tank top or loose-fitting pants and a t-shirt. Remember, the key is to feel at ease in your body as you flow through the poses.

4. Gather Props (Optional):

Depending on your preferences and needs, you may want to have some props on hand to enhance your practice. Consider using a yoga block or a folded blanket to support certain poses or provide extra cushioning. Props can help modify poses to accommodate your body's unique needs and enhance your overall experience.

5. Set Intentions:

Take a moment to set your intentions for your chair yoga practice. Whether it's to improve flexibility, build strength, or simply unwind and relax, clarifying your goals will guide your focus and motivation throughout the session. Visualize yourself achieving these intentions and embrace a positive mindset as you begin your practice.

By taking the time to prepare your space and mindset, you set yourself up for a rewarding and fulfilling chair yoga experience. Remember to listen to your body, honor your limitations, and enjoy the journey towards improved health and well-being.

In the next chapter, we'll dive into the foundations of chair yoga and explore basic poses to get you started on your weight loss journey. Get ready to strengthen your body, calm your mind, and transform your life with chair yoga.

Chapter 3: Chair Yoga Pose: A Comprehensive Guide to Weight Loss Chair Sun Salutations

In this chapter, we'll explore a series of chair yoga poses specifically designed to promote weight loss and overall wellness. These Chair Sun Salutations offer a dynamic sequence that targets key muscle groups, improves circulation, and boosts metabolism. Let's dive into each pose in detail:

1. Seated Mountain Pose:

Begin by sitting tall in your chair with your feet flat on the floor, hip-width apart. Ground down through your sit bones and lengthen through your spine. Engage your core muscles and roll your shoulders back, opening your chest. Extend your arms alongside your body, palms facing forward. Take several deep breaths, feeling grounded and rooted like a mountain.

2. Seated Forward Bend:

From Seated Mountain Pose, inhale as you reach your arms overhead. Exhale, hinge at your hips, and slowly fold forward, bringing your hands towards the floor or your shins. Keep your spine long and your neck relaxed. Hold the stretch for a few breaths, feeling a gentle release in your hamstrings and lower back.

3. Chair Warrior Pose:

Come back to a seated position with your feet flat on the floor. Extend your right leg out to the side, keeping your left foot grounded. Bend your left knee and engage your core as you lift your arms overhead, palms facing each other. Sink into your left hip, feeling a stretch through your inner thigh and groin. Hold for a few breaths, then switch sides.

4. Seated Spinal Twist:

Return to a neutral seated position with both feet flat on the floor. Place your right hand on the outside of your left knee and your left hand on the back of the chair. Inhale to lengthen your spine, then exhale as you twist gently to the left, looking over your left shoulder. Keep your hips grounded and your spine tall. Hold for a few breaths, then repeat on the other side.

5. Chair Pigeon Pose:

Sit on the edge of your chair with your feet flat on the floor. Cross your right ankle over your left knee, flexing your right foot. Keep your spine tall as you hinge forward from your hips, leading with your chest. You should feel a stretch in your right outer hip and glute.

Hold for a few breaths, then switch sides.

6. Chair Cat-Cow Stretch:

Come back to a neutral seated position with your hands resting on your knees. Inhale as you arch your back, lifting your chest and tilting your pelvis forward (Cow Pose). Exhale as you round your spine, tucking your chin to your chest and drawing your belly button towards your spine (Cat Pose). Flow smoothly between these two poses, synchronizing your breath with your movement.

Practice these Chair Sun Salutations regularly to improve flexibility, build strength, and support your weight loss journey. Remember to listen to your body and modify the poses as needed to suit your individual needs and abilities. Enjoy the benefits of chair yoga as you work towards achieving your health and wellness goals.

Chapter 4: Chair Yoga Exercises: Weight Loss Movements and Methods Morning Routine

Welcome to Chapter 4 of "Chair Yoga for Weight Loss: Two in One". In this chapter, we will explore a morning routine specifically designed to kickstart your metabolism, energize your body, and set a positive tone for the day ahead. Get ready to embrace the power of chair yoga as we incorporate dynamic movements and effective techniques to support your weight loss journey.

1. Sunrise Salutation:

  - Begin seated comfortably on your chair with your feet flat on the floor and your spine tall.

- Inhale as you raise your arms overhead, reaching towards the sky.

- Exhale as you twist gently to the right, placing your left hand on your right knee and your right hand on the back of the chair.

- Inhale as you return to center, then exhale as you twist to the left, placing your right hand on your left knee and your left hand on the back of the chair.

- Repeat this twisting motion several times, flowing with your breath and warming up your spine.

2. Midday Stretch Break:

- As the day progresses and tension builds, take a moment to pause and reset with a midday stretch break.

- Stand up from your chair and stretch your arms overhead, reaching towards the ceiling.

- Take a deep breath in and exhale as you fold forward, reaching towards your toes or the floor.

- Hold this forward fold for a few breaths, allowing your spine to lengthen and your hamstrings to release.

- Slowly roll back up to a standing position and return to your chair feeling refreshed and rejuvenated.

3. Morning Flow:

- Sit tall in your chair with your feet hip-width apart and your hands resting on your knees.

- Inhale as you lift your arms overhead, stretching towards the sky.

- Exhale as you twist gently to the right, bringing your left hand to your right knee and your right hand to the back of the chair.

- Inhale to lengthen your spine, then exhale to deepen the twist.

- Hold this twist for a few breaths, feeling the gentle compression in your abdomen.

- Inhale as you return to center, then exhale as you twist to the left, repeating the same sequence on the opposite side.

- Flow through this sequence several times, moving with your breath and awakening your body.

4. Evening Flow: Calm:

- As the day comes to a close, transition into a calming evening flow to unwind and relax.

- Sit comfortably in your chair with your feet grounded and your palms resting on your thighs.

- Close your eyes and take several deep breaths, allowing yourself to let go of any tension or stress from the day.

- With each inhale, imagine breathing in peace and serenity. With each exhale, release any worries or distractions.

- Spend a few minutes in this quiet, meditative state, savoring the stillness and calmness within. When you feel ready, gently open your eyes and carry this sense of tranquility with you as you prepare for restful sleep.

Chapter 5: Chair Yoga Adjustments and Supplements: Tailoring Positions to All Ability Levels

In this chapter, we'll delve into the art of adapting chair yoga poses to accommodate individuals of all ability levels. Whether you're a beginner just starting your yoga journey or someone with physical limitations, these adjustments and supplements will ensure that everyone can reap the benefits of chair yoga for weight loss.

1. Understanding Individual Needs: Before diving into the practice, it's essential to assess the unique needs of each practitioner. Take into account any physical limitations, injuries, or health conditions that may require modifications to the poses.

2. Use of Props: Props such as yoga blocks, straps, and cushions can be invaluable tools for making poses more accessible. For example, using a block or cushion to elevate the hips can provide added support and stability in seated poses.

3. Chair Variations: Experiment with different types of chairs to find one that best suits your needs. Some individuals may prefer a chair with armrests for added support, while others may find a folding chair or stability ball more comfortable.

4. Gentle Modifications: For beginners or those with limited mobility, gentle modifications can make poses more approachable. For example, in seated forward folds, encourage students to bend their knees slightly to reduce strain on the lower back.

5. Breath Awareness: Emphasize the importance of breath awareness throughout the practice. Encourage students to focus on deep, mindful breathing to enhance relaxation and reduce stress.

6. Seated Sun Salutations: Explore modified versions of traditional sun salutations that can be performed entirely in a seated position. These flowing sequences offer a full-body workout while promoting flexibility and circulation.

7. Standing Support: For individuals who are able, incorporate standing poses with the support of a chair or wall. Standing poses like tree pose or warrior variations can build strength and balance while improving posture.

8. Visualization and Affirmations: Integrate visualization techniques and positive affirmations into the practice to enhance motivation and mental focus. Encourage students to visualize themselves achieving their weight loss goals and affirm their strength and resilience.

9. Guided Relaxation: Conclude each session with a guided relaxation or meditation to promote deep relaxation and stress relief. Use calming imagery and soothing language to guide students into a state of inner peace and tranquility.

By incorporating these adjustments and supplements into your chair yoga practice, you can create a safe, inclusive environment where everyone can experience the transformative benefits of yoga for weight loss. Remember to always prioritize the individual needs and comfort of your students, and encourage them to listen to their bodies and modify as needed. With patience, compassion, and dedication, chair yoga can become a powerful tool for achieving your fitness goals and cultivating overall well-being.

In the next chapter, we'll explore specific chair yoga sequences designed to target key areas of the body for weight loss and toning. Get ready to sweat, stretch, and strengthen as we dive deeper into the practice of chair yoga for weight loss.

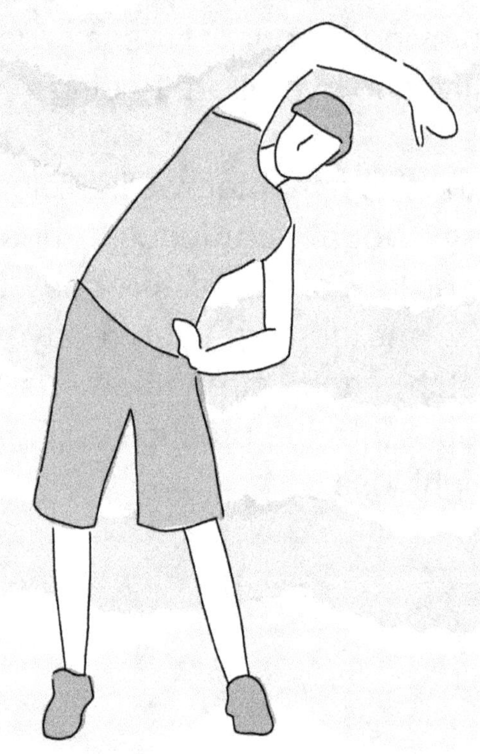

Chapter 6: Breathing Techniques: Incorporating Pranayama for Improved Results

Welcome to Chapter 6 of "Chair Yoga for Weight Loss: Two in One". In this chapter, we will explore the profound impact that breathing techniques, known as pranayama, can have on enhancing your chair yoga practice and achieving your weight loss goals. Pranayama, the ancient yogic art of breath control, offers a powerful tool for promoting physical, mental, and emotional well-being. By incorporating pranayama into your chair yoga routine, you can amplify the benefits of your practice and accelerate your progress towards weight loss and overall wellness.

1. Understanding Pranayama: Pranayama techniques involve conscious manipulation of the breath to regulate the flow of prana, or life force energy, within the body. By harnessing the power of the breath, we can influence our physiological functions, calm the mind, and cultivate inner awareness.

2. Benefits of Pranayama for Weight Loss: Pranayama techniques can play a significant role in supporting weight loss efforts. Deep breathing exercises stimulate the metabolism, improve digestion, and promote detoxification of the body. Additionally, certain pranayama practices can help reduce stress and emotional eating, leading to more mindful food choices and better weight management.

3. Incorporating Pranayama into Your Chair Yoga Practice: Begin by finding a comfortable seated position in your chair, with your feet flat on the ground and your spine tall. Close your eyes and take a few deep breaths to center yourself. Then, explore the following pranayama techniques:

Deep Belly Breathing: Place one hand on your abdomen and the other on your chest. Inhale deeply through your nose, allowing your belly to expand as you fill your lungs with air. Exhale slowly through your mouth, drawing your navel towards your spine. Repeat this cycle several times, focusing on the sensation of your breath moving in and out of your body.

Alternate Nostril Breathing (Nadi Shodhana): Close your right nostril with your right thumb and inhale deeply through your left nostril. Then, close your left nostril with your ring finger and exhale through your right nostril. Inhale through your right nostril, then switch to exhaling through your left nostril. Continue this alternating pattern for several rounds, feeling the calming effect of balanced breathing.

Kapalabhati (Skull Shining Breath): Sit up tall and take a deep breath in. Then, forcefully exhale through your nose by contracting your abdominal muscles. Allow the inhalation to happen passively. Repeat this rapid exhalation-inhalation cycle for 30-60 seconds, focusing on the sensation of energy moving through your body.

4. Practicing Mindful Breathing: As you engage in pranayama exercises, cultivate a sense of mindfulness and presence. Pay attention to the quality of your breath and observe any sensations or thoughts that arise without judgment. By anchoring your awareness to the present moment, you can deepen your connection to your body and enhance the efficacy of your chair yoga practice.

Incorporate these pranayama techniques into your daily chair yoga routine to supercharge your weight loss journey and promote holistic well-being. As you harness the power of your breath, you will discover a newfound sense of vitality, balance, and inner harmony. Stay tuned for Chapter 7, where we will delve into the importance of relaxation and mindfulness in supporting sustainable weight loss goals.

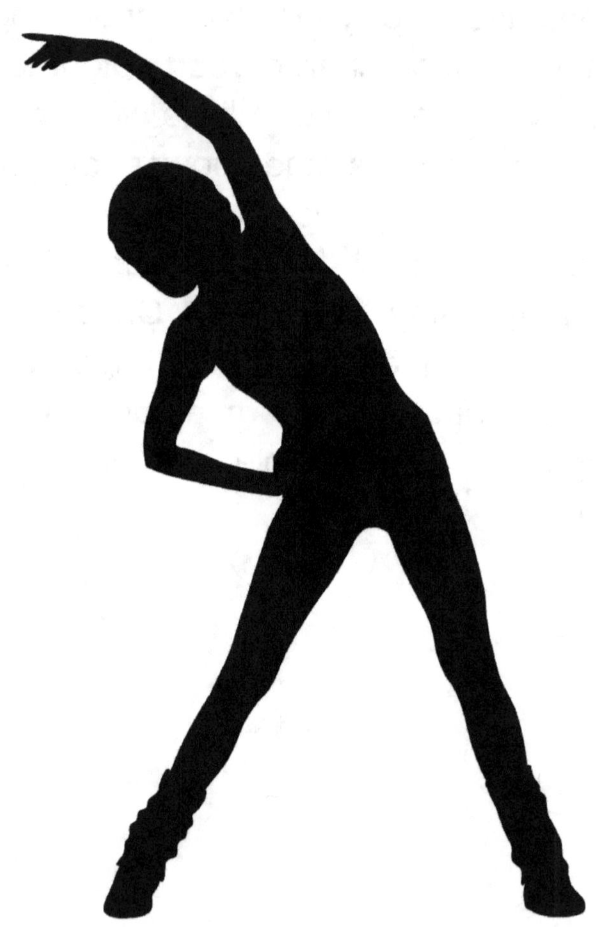

Chapter 7: Mindful Eating: Integrating Yoga Philosophy with Nutrition

Welcome to Chapter 7 of "Chair Yoga for Weight Loss: Two in One". In this chapter, we'll explore the concept of mindful eating and how it can complement your chair yoga practice to support your weight loss journey.

Yoga Philosophy and Nutrition:
Yoga teaches us to be present in the moment and to cultivate awareness of our body, mind, and spirit. This same philosophy can be applied to our eating habits, leading to greater enjoyment of food and improved overall well-being.

Mindful Eating Basics:
Mindful eating is about paying attention to the sensory experience of eating, including the taste, texture, and aroma of food. It involves slowing down, savoring each bite, and listening to your body's hunger and fullness cues.

Here are some tips for practicing mindful eating:

1. Eat slowly: Take your time to chew each bite thoroughly and fully experience the flavors of your food.

2. Use all your senses: Notice the colors, smells, and textures of your food before taking a bite.

3. Listen to your body: Pay attention to your hunger and fullness signals, and eat only until you are satisfied, not overly full.

4. Avoid distractions: Turn off the TV, put away your phone, and focus solely on the act of eating.

5. Express gratitude: Before you begin your meal, take a moment to express gratitude for the nourishment it provides.

Integrating Mindful Eating with Chair Yoga:

Chair yoga can enhance your mindful eating practice by helping you develop greater body awareness and self-control. Incorporate the following chair yoga poses and techniques into your meals to promote mindfulness and aid in weight loss:

1. Seated Spinal Twist: Sit tall in your chair and gently twist your torso to one side, placing one hand on the opposite knee and the other hand on the back of the chair. Take a few deep breaths as you twist, then repeat on the other side. This pose aids in digestion and can help alleviate bloating.

2. Seated Forward Bend: Sit at the edge of your chair with your feet hip-width apart. Inhale to lengthen your spine, then exhale to fold forward from your hips, reaching your hands towards your feet or the floor. Hold for a few breaths, then slowly return to an upright position. This pose stimulates the digestive organs and can improve metabolism.

3. Mindful Eating Meditation: Before you begin your meal, take a few moments to close your eyes and bring your attention to your breath. Notice any sensations in your body and any thoughts or emotions that arise. As you eat, continue to focus on your breath and the sensory experience of eating. If your mind wanders, gently bring it back to the present moment.

By integrating mindful eating with your chair yoga practice, you can cultivate a healthier relationship with food, improve digestion, and support your weight loss goals. Take the time to savor each meal and nourish your body and soul with love and awareness.

In the next chapter, we'll explore how chair yoga can help reduce stress and emotional eating. Until then, remember to eat mindfully, move with intention, and embrace the journey towards holistic well-being.

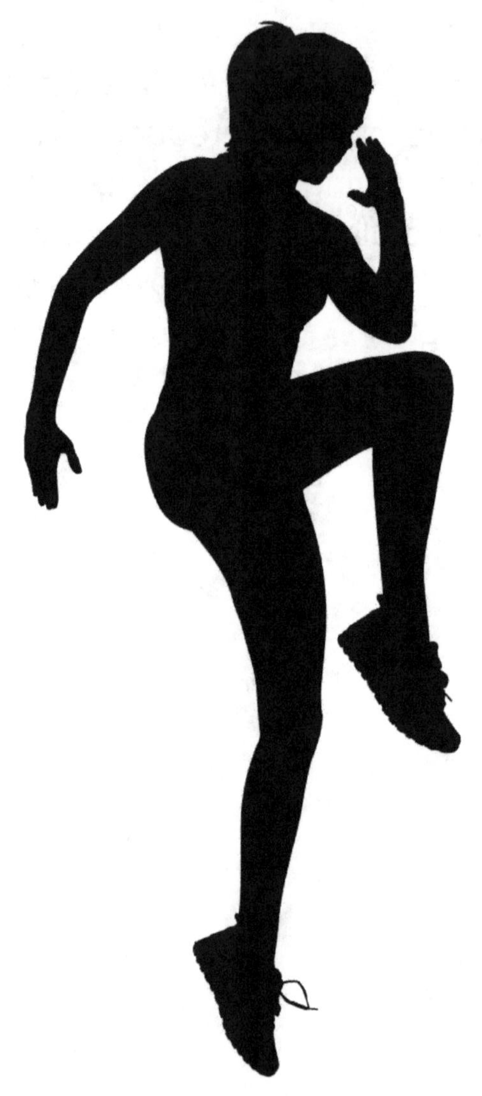

Chapter 8: Combining Chair Yoga with Other Exercises to Create a Fitness Programme That Is Well-Balanced

In this chapter, we will explore how to integrate chair yoga seamlessly with other exercises to create a holistic fitness program that promotes overall well-being and weight loss. While chair yoga offers numerous benefits on its own, combining it with other forms of exercise can enhance results and provide a well-rounded approach to fitness.

1. Understanding the Benefits of Cross-Training:

- Cross-training involves incorporating a variety of exercises into your workout routine to target different muscle groups, prevent boredom, and reduce the risk of overuse injuries.

- By combining chair yoga with other exercises, such as cardiovascular activities, strength training, and flexibility exercises, you can maximize the benefits of each workout session.

2. Designing Your Fitness Programme:

- Begin by identifying your fitness goals and assessing your current level of fitness.

- Incorporate chair yoga sessions into your weekly schedule, aiming for at least two to three sessions per week.

- Choose complementary exercises that align with your goals, such as walking, swimming, cycling, or aerobics for cardiovascular health, and resistance training or bodyweight exercises for strength.

- Schedule rest days to allow your body to recover and prevent burnout.

3. Sample Fitness Programme:
- **Monday:** Chair Yoga for Weight Loss session focusing on core strength and flexibility.
- **Tuesday:** 30-minute brisk walk or cycling session for cardiovascular health.
- **Wednesday:** Chair Yoga for Weight Loss session targeting upper body strength and balance.
- **Thursday:** Resistance training or bodyweight exercises for muscle building and toning.
- **Friday:** Chair Yoga for Weight Loss session emphasizing relaxation and stress reduction.
- **Saturday:** Rest day or gentle activities such as swimming or tai chi.
- **Sunday:** Long walk or hike to improve endurance and promote mental clarity.

4. Tips for Success:

- Listen to your body and modify exercises as needed to accommodate any limitations or injuries.

- Stay hydrated and fuel your body with nutritious foods to support your workouts. Incorporate mindfulness techniques from chair yoga, such as deep breathing and meditation, into your other exercises to enhance focus and reduce stress. Keep track of your progress and celebrate your achievements along the way.

By combining chair yoga with other exercises, you can create a fitness program that is both effective and enjoyable. Experiment with different activities to find what works best for you, and remember to prioritize consistency and balance in your approach to fitness. With dedication and perseverance, you can achieve your weight loss goals and improve your overall health and well-being.

Chapter 9: Tracking Your Progress: Setting Goals and Keeping an Eye on Outcomes

Congratulations on making it to Chapter 9 of "Chair Yoga for Weight Loss: Two in One"! By now, you've likely experienced the transformative power of chair yoga in both your physical and mental well-being. As you continue on your journey towards a healthier you, it's essential to track your progress, set realistic goals, and stay focused on achieving outcomes that align with your aspirations.

Setting SMART Goals

When it comes to achieving your fitness goals, specificity is key. That's where SMART goals come in. SMART stands for Specific, Measurable, Achievable, Relevant, and Time-bound. Let's break it down:

1. Specific: Clearly define what you want to accomplish. Instead of saying, "I want to lose weight," specify how much weight you aim to lose and in what timeframe.

2. Measurable: Your goals should be quantifiable so you can track your progress. For example, "I want to lose 10 pounds in two months."

3. Achievable: Be realistic about what you can accomplish. Setting overly ambitious goals can lead to frustration and burnout. Start with small, achievable milestones and build from there.

4. Relevant: Your goals should align with your overall objectives and values. If your main focus is weight loss, set goals related to calorie intake, physical activity, and mindfulness practices that support this objective.

5. Time-bound: Give yourself a deadline to work towards. Having a timeframe creates a sense of urgency and helps you stay motivated.

Tracking Your Progress

Once you've set your goals, it's crucial to monitor your progress regularly. Here are some effective ways to track your journey:

1. Keep a Journal: Record your daily chair yoga sessions, meals, water intake, and any thoughts or feelings related to your progress. Reflecting on your journal entries can provide valuable insights into your habits and behaviors.

2. Use Technology: There are numerous fitness apps and wearable devices available that can help you track your physical activity, calorie intake, and weight loss progress. Find one that works for you and integrate it into your routine.

3. Measurements and Photos: Take measurements of your body (such as waist circumference, hip circumference, and body fat percentage) and progress photos at regular intervals. Seeing tangible results can be incredibly motivating.

4. Celebrate Milestones: Acknowledge and celebrate your achievements along the way, whether it's reaching a weight loss milestone, mastering a challenging yoga pose, or noticing improvements in your flexibility and stamina.

Adjusting Your Approach

As you track your progress, you may encounter obstacles or setbacks. Remember that setbacks are a natural part of any journey, and they provide valuable learning opportunities. If you find that you're not progressing as quickly as you'd like, don't be afraid to reassess your goals and adjust your approach accordingly. Be flexible and open-minded, and don't hesitate to seek support from friends, family, or a healthcare professional if needed.

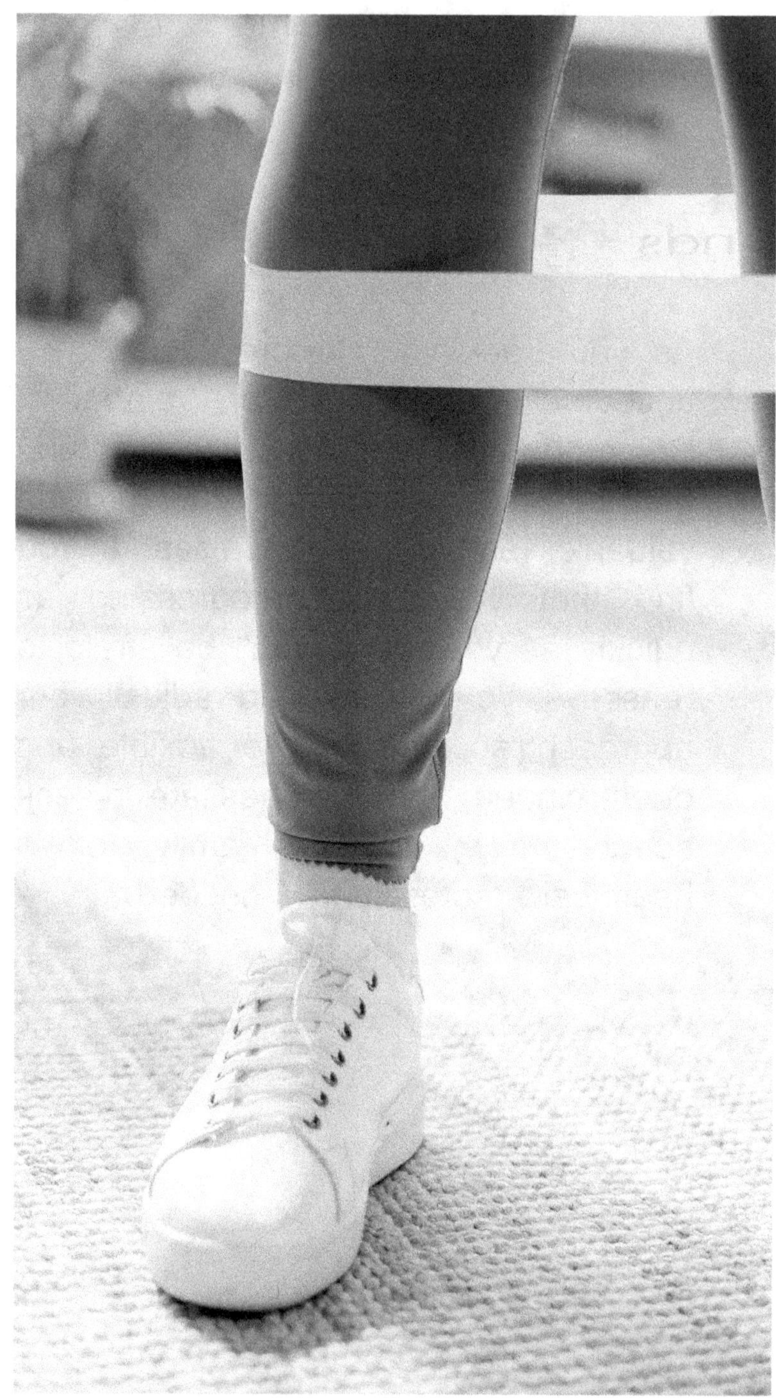

Chapter 10: Frequently Asked Questions (FAQs) About Chair Yoga and Weight Loss

As you embark on your journey with chair yoga for weight loss, you may have questions about the practice, its benefits, and how it can help you achieve your fitness goals. In this chapter, we'll address some of the most common questions to help you gain a deeper understanding of chair yoga and its role in weight loss.

1. What is chair yoga, and how does it differ from traditional yoga?

Chair yoga is a modified form of yoga that incorporates the use of a chair to support and assist in performing yoga poses. It is especially beneficial for individuals with limited mobility or those who find it challenging to practice yoga on a mat. Chair yoga focuses on gentle movements, stretches, and breathing exercises, making it accessible to people of all fitness levels.

2. Can chair yoga help with weight loss?

Yes, chair yoga can be an effective tool for weight loss when combined with a healthy diet and lifestyle. While chair yoga may not burn as many calories as high-intensity workouts, it can still contribute to weight loss by increasing metabolism, improving muscle tone, and promoting overall well-being. Additionally, chair yoga helps reduce stress and emotional eating, which are common barriers to weight loss.

3. How often should I practice chair yoga for weight loss?

The frequency of your chair yoga practice depends on your individual goals, schedule, and fitness level. Ideally, aim to practice chair yoga for at least 20-30 minutes, 3-5 times per week to see noticeable results. Consistency is key, so try to establish a regular practice routine that works for you.

4. Are there specific poses or sequences that are best for weight loss?

While any form of physical activity can contribute to weight loss, certain chair yoga poses and sequences are particularly effective for targeting specific areas of the body and promoting calorie burning. Poses that engage multiple muscle groups, such as chair squats, leg lifts, and seated twists, are great choices for toning and strengthening the body. Additionally, incorporating dynamic movements and flowing sequences can help elevate the heart rate and increase energy expenditure.

5. Can chair yoga help with stress-related eating and emotional wellness?

Absolutely! Chair yoga is not only beneficial for physical fitness but also for mental and emotional well-being. The mindfulness techniques and breathing exercises practiced in chair yoga help reduce stress, anxiety, and emotional eating patterns. By cultivating a sense of calm and inner peace, chair yoga empowers you to make healthier choices and maintain a balanced relationship with food. By incorporating chair yoga into your weight loss journey, you can enhance your physical fitness, improve your mental well-being, and achieve lasting results. Experiment with different poses, sequences, and mindfulness practices to find what works best for you. Remember, consistency, patience, and self-compassion are key as you progress on your path to wellness.

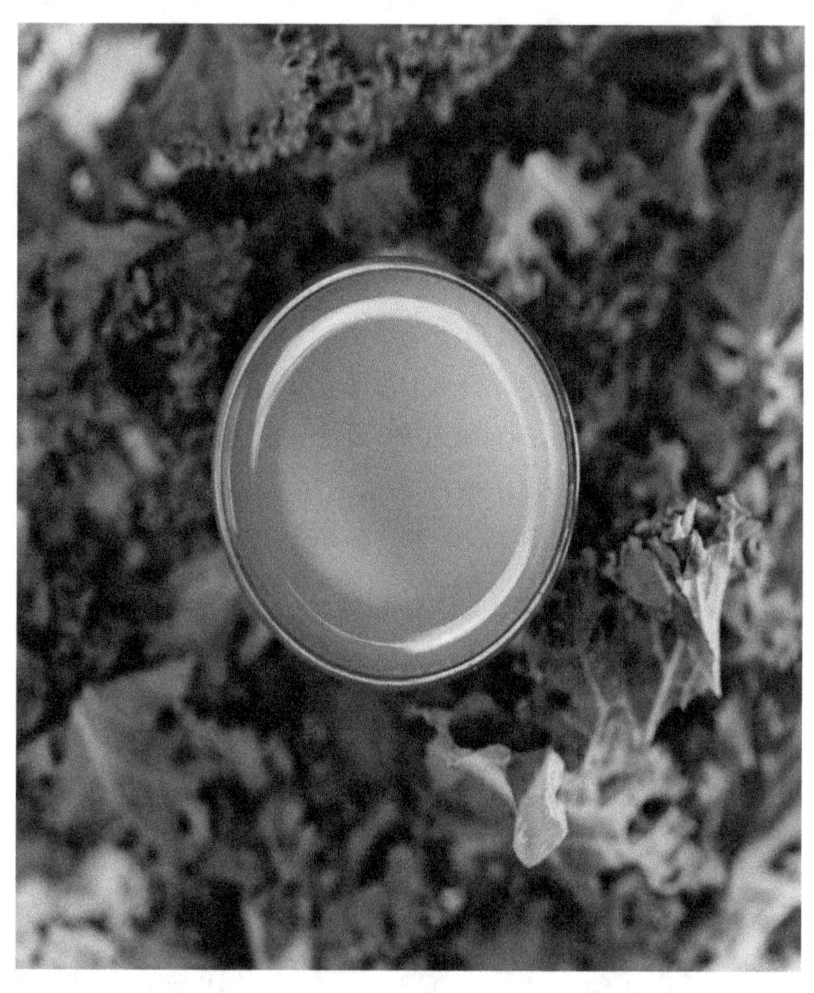

Chapter 11: Bonus Recipes for Healthy Living

In this chapter, we're diving into the world of culinary delights with a collection of bonus recipes to complement your chair yoga practice. From refreshing drinks to nutritious salads and satisfying snacks, these recipes are designed to nourish your body and support your weight loss journey.

1. Vibrant Drinks:

Kickstart your day with a burst of energy and vitality by incorporating these vibrant drink recipes into your routine:

- Green Goddess Smoothie:
INGREDIENTS:
- 1 cup spinach leaves
- 1/2 cucumber, peeled and chopped
- 1/2 green apple, cored and chopped
- 1/2 lemon, juiced
- 1/2 inch piece of ginger, peeled
- 1/2 cup coconut water
- Ice cubes (optional)

INSTRUCTIONS:

1. Combine all ingredients in a blender and blend until smooth.

2. Add ice cubes if desired and blend again until well combined.

3. Pour into a glass and enjoy this refreshing green goddess smoothie packed with nutrients and flavor.

– Berry Blast Juice:

INGREDIENTS:

- 1 cup mixed berries (such as strawberries, blueberries, and raspberries)
- 1/2 cup coconut water
- 1 tablespoon honey or maple syrup (optional)
- Ice cubes (optional)

INSTRUCTIONS:

1. Place the mixed berries and coconut water in a blender.

2. Add honey or maple syrup if using, and blend until smooth.

3. If desired, add ice cubes and blend again until well combined.

4. Pour into a glass and savor the refreshing burst of berry goodness.

2. Healthy Salads:

Elevate your mealtime with these vibrant and nutrient-packed salad recipes:

- Mediterranean Quinoa Salad:
INGREDIENTS:

- 1 cup cooked quinoa
- 1 cup cherry tomatoes, halved
- 1/2 cucumber, diced
- 1/4 cup Kalamata olives, pitted and sliced
- 1/4 cup crumbled feta cheese
- 2 tablespoons chopped fresh parsley
- 1 tablespoon extra virgin olive oil
- 1 tablespoon lemon juice
- Salt and pepper to taste

INSTRUCTIONS:

1. In a large bowl, combine the cooked quinoa, cherry tomatoes, cucumber, olives, feta cheese, and parsley.

2. Drizzle with olive oil and lemon juice, and season with salt and pepper to taste.

3. Toss gently to combine, then serve and enjoy this Mediterranean-inspired quinoa salad bursting with flavor and nutrients.

- Crunchy Kale Salad:
INGREDIENTS:

- 4 cups chopped kale leaves
- 1/2 cup shredded carrots
- 1/4 cup sliced almonds
- 1/4 cup dried cranberries
- 2 tablespoons lemon juice
- 1 tablespoon extra virgin olive oil
- 1 teaspoon honey or maple syrup
- Salt and pepper to taste

INSTRUCTIONS:

1. In a large bowl, combine the chopped kale, shredded carrots, sliced almonds, and dried cranberries.

2. In a small bowl, whisk together the lemon juice, olive oil, honey or maple syrup, salt, and pepper.

3. Pour the dressing over the salad and toss gently to coat.

4. Let the salad marinate for a few minutes before serving, allowing the flavors to meld together. Enjoy this crunchy kale salad as a nutritious and satisfying meal or side dish.

3. Delectable and Light Snacks:

Satisfy your cravings with these guilt-free snack recipes that are both delicious and nutritious:

- **Avocado Toast Bites:**
  INGREDIENTS:
    - 4 slices whole grain bread, toasted
    - 1 ripe avocado
    - Cherry tomatoes, sliced
    - Red pepper flakes (optional)
    - Sea salt (optional)

  INSTRUCTIONS:
    1. Mash the ripe avocado in a bowl until smooth.
    2. Spread the mashed avocado evenly onto the toasted bread slices.
    3. Top each toast with sliced cherry tomatoes.

4. Sprinkle with red pepper flakes and sea salt if desired.

5. Cut each toast into bite-sized pieces and serve as a tasty and nutritious snack option.

- Greek Yogurt Dip with Veggie Sticks:

INGREDIENTS:
- 1 cup Greek yogurt
- 1 tablespoon lemon juice
- 1 clove garlic, minced
- 1 tablespoon chopped fresh dill
- Assorted vegetable sticks (such as carrots, cucumbers, and bell peppers)

INSTRUCTIONS:

1. In a small bowl, mix together the Greek yogurt, lemon juice, minced garlic, and chopped fresh dill.

2. Season with salt and pepper to taste.

3. Serve the Greek yogurt dip with assorted vegetable sticks for a satisfying

and nutritious snack option that's perfect for dipping.

Thank you for choosing to embark on this journey with me. I am honored to be your guide as we explore the transformative power of chair yoga together.

Chapter 12: Conclusion Thoughts: Chair Yoga – Embracing Well-being

As we approach the conclusion of "Chair Yoga for Weight Loss: Two in One," it is fitting to reflect on our transformative journey together. In this e-book, we've looked at the strong link between chair yoga and weight loss and discovered how this gentle yet effective practice can enhance overall health and physical fitness.

In our fast-paced environment, it's easy to get caught up in the pursuit of external goals, such as getting more muscle or losing weight. While these are certainly important objectives, true well-being extends much beyond physical attractiveness. It entails cultivating a sense of harmony and balance within oneself as well as forging a solid connection between the mind, body, and spirit.

Chair yoga offers a path to overall wellness by encouraging us to embrace our bodies for what they are—amazing machines with limitless potential. By engaging in mindful movement, aware breathing, and self-compassion exercises, we may access our inner resilience and strength, which will enable us to find strength and fulfilment in the present moment.

As this e-book has taught us, chair yoga is about more than just the poses we do and the calories we burn. It's about learning to love and accept who we are right now and about honouring ourselves for who we are. It's about letting go of judgement and embracing gratitude for the incredible gift of life.

Once you turn the page and continue your chair yoga adventure, never forget to approach each practice with an open heart and a loving spirit. Recognise the wisdom of your body, and treat its needs and limitations with kindness and affection. Above all, never forget that you are worthy of acceptance, affection, and pleasure in your current form.

It is my aim that the practices and teachings found in this e-book can support you on your path to greater wellbeing, completeness, and health. May you constantly practice self-care for your body, mind, and soul with the elegance and wisdom of a real yogi.

Thank you for joining me on this path of self-discovery and development. Through your chair yoga practice, I wish you many years of strength, calm, and rich well-being.

With gratitude and warm regards,

The author of the book "Chair Yoga for Weight Loss: Two in One" is

[Dr. Jerry Taylor].